THE GIANTS OF GERIATRICS

The Chair which I have the honour to inaugurate today is the eighth Chair of Geriatric Medicine to be established at Universities in the United Kingdom. Its foundation is a tribute to the importance now attached to the education of the doctors of today and tomorrow in the emerging specialty of geriatric medicine; and to the imaginative contribution of generous private benefactors to the field of medical education. The Charitable Trust established by Sir Charles Hayward has contributed to many fields of endeavour and of help to the aged, and it is appropriate that Sir Charles's name should be permanently linked with the Medical School which serves the West Midlands where so much of his life's work was done.

I have chosen as my title "The Giants of Geriatrics". These **giants are the afflictions which beset many people in advanced** old age. They are:—

Immobility, Instability, Incontinence and Intellectual Impairment.

They pose an ever-growing threat to the comfort and happiness of old people and their helpers, and to the efficiency and integrity of the health and social services.

I define the "giants" as follows:—

Immobility is the inability to walk safely and without human support at least as far as the nearest toilet.

Instability is the tendency to lose balance and fall.

Incontinence is the involuntary passage of urine and/or faeces.

Intellectual Impairment implies a loss of the functions of the brain of such severity that safe and independent living become impossible.

The presence of one or more of these symptoms creates a state of *"dependence"*, defined as the subject's inability to provide for himself the basic needs of food, warmth, cleanliness and safety at an acceptable standard.

The "Giants" have in common the following attributes:—

(1) They are of multiple causation.
(2) They rob the victim of his independence.
(3) They are not life-threatening.
(4) They do not readily respond to simple therapeutic measures.

It is these attributes which make them such baffling and demanding challenges to our system of medical care.

1

These symptoms are common, and their frequency increases with age. In a recent survey of three communities in the West of Scotland (Isaacs and Neville, 1976) the prevalence of the four symptoms was as follows:—

TABLE I

Estimated Prevalence of "Giants of Geriatrics"

Symptom	Estimated prevalence per 1,000 of age-group		
	65–74	75–84	85 and Over
Immobility	23	58	166
Instability	10	10	29
Incontinence	12	34	118
Intellectual Impairment	7	39	79

Data from Isaacs and Neville, 1976.

In the same study the prevalence of dependence was found to be closely related to age, but not to sex, social class, family structure, living arrangements or any other variable studied. In the age group 65 to 74, 4% of the population were dependent. The corresponding figures for the other age-groups were 10% of those aged 75 to 84 and 24% of those aged 85 and over. If these figures were to be applied to the population of England and Wales as in 1971, the following rough estimates of the national prevalence of these symptoms would be obtained:—

A quarter of a million people would be immobile, seventy thousand liable to fall, one hundred and sixty thousand incontinent and one hundred and thirty thousand suffering from severe intellectual impairment.

TABLE II

Estimated number of victims of "Giants of Geriatrics" in England and Wales, 1971

Symptom	Number in age-group with symptom (thousands)			
	65–74	75–84	85 and Over	All aged 65 and Over
Immobility	97	107	70	274
Instability	42	18	12	72
Incontinence	50	63	50	163
Intellectual Impairment	30	72	33	135

In the Scottish study, for every subject with immobility who was in hospital there were 2 with the same degree of disability at home; for every 2 incontinent subjects in hospital there were 3 at home; and for every 3 with significant intellectual impairment in hospital there were 4 with a similar degree of abnormality at home.

The extent to which families cared for dependent old people is illustrated in the following figures. Of dependent subjects who lived alone three-quarters were in hospital; of those who lived with a spouse or other old people one in three were in hospital, and of those who lived with their children one in eight were in hospital.

In the last three decades of the present century the population will age, and this trend will be greatest amongst the very old.

TABLE III

Projected Population Changes in England and Wales

(Registrar General's Statistical Review)

Age-group	Population 1971 (thousands)	Estimated Population 2001 (thousands)	Percentage Change
65–74	4229	4041	- 5
75–84	1849	2493	+35
85 and Over	423	653	+54
All aged 65 and Over	6501	7187	+11

There will actually be a small drop towards the end of the century in the numbers aged 65 to 74, reflecting the fall in birth rate which followed the First World War. But the 75 to 84 age group will increase by one-third, and the 85 and over age-group by one-half.

If the prevalence of these symptoms by age-group remains the same—and there is little prospect at present of a major reduction in any of them—then there will be a disproportionate increase, with the growth of the elderly population, in the number suffering from the symptoms of dependency. (See Table IV). Thus for example, for every three intellectually impaired old persons today, there will be a fourth one in 2001; for every six liable to fall there will be a seventh. The greater part of the increase in numbers of these dependent people will be among those aged 85 and over.

A characteristic feature of the "Giants of Geriatrics" is the dependence of their victims on other people's efforts to care for them. The population survey already referred to confirmed the findings of a previous study of geriatric patients (Isaacs, 1972) which showed that the main burden of caring at home was borne by relatives in the age-group 45–64. This age-group also forms a substantial proportion of those working with old people in the hospital and domiciliary services. The main need for care comes from patients aged 75 and over. A measure of the potential availability of care for the aged is the ratio of the population aged 45 to 64 to that aged 75 and over. Table V gives the values for this "index of geriatric care" in the United Kingdom during this century. The figure has fallen from a ratio of 12:1 as recently as 1931 to 5:1 in 1971, and it is anticipated that it will fall further to 3.5:1 in 1991.

It is clear that a major effort must now be directed towards the prevention and treatment of the four "giant" symptoms. One reason for delay in so doing in the past is suggested by a survey which my colleagues and I undertook in 1968 (Isaacs, 1972) in which we compared the characteristics of patients aged 65 and over who were admitted to the medical wards of a teaching hospital with others of the same age group admitted to a geriatric unit serving the same area. The main difference between the two groups was that whereas two-thirds of those entering the geriatric wards had two or more of the symptoms of dependency, two-thirds of those admitted to the medical wards had none of these symptoms. (See Table IV).* The probable reason was that, historically, acute medical units had erected barriers against the admission of aged patients suffering from these symptoms, and thus had perpetuated a situation in which medical students and young doctors failed to have their attention directed towards an important area of medical need. Much has changed since 1968, and general medical wards today experience, on a much larger scale, the admission of this group of patients. It is towards the elucidation of the causes, prevention and treatment of these four symptoms that I shall devote the remainder of this lecture.

IMMOBILITY

The major causes of impaired mobility in the elderly are:—

(1) Diseases of the joints, especially osteoarthrosis of the hips and knees.
(2) Trauma, especially fractures of the upper end of the femur.
(3) Amputation of the lower limbs.
(4) Stroke
(5) Parkinsonism
(6) Other less well defined cerebral disturbances, such as apraxia of gait (Adams, 1974).
(7) Other neurological conditions, e.g. peripheral neuropathy, multiple sclerosis, etc.
(8) Defects of the feet.

Often the restoration of mobility depends less on the primary disease than on the patient's general physical and mental state, the co-existence of obesity, cardiorespiratory and other disorders

* In this study a fifth presenting symptom was included, namely "stroke".

5

and the intellectual capacity and will to participate in active treatment. Environmental factors, such as the type of house and the attitudes of relatives, play a further important part.

Restoration of mobility has three objectives:—

Independence in self-propulsion;
Independence in transfers;
Independence in ambulation.

Of these, the second is crucial.
Transfers i.e. the ability to move safely from bed to chair, from chair to wheelchair, and from wheelchair to toilet are as important to ambulation as is take-off and landing to flying. No-one would take up an aeroplane off a potato field, yet many frail old people, at home and in hospital, have to transfer from a high bed to a low chair, or from a high wheelchair to a low toilet, in ill-fitting slippers and on poor floor surfaces, at the hands of staff or relatives who have received little instruction in the appropriate methods. The achievement of safe transfer requires little knowledge but much organisation. The one is there, the other is not, and it must be supplied.

Self-propulsion offers the prospect of independent locomotion early in rehabilitation. Most immobile patients can and should be trained to use a wheelchair during the early stages of rehabilitation, and should be weaned from it as the will and capacity for independent mobility is strengthened. Those who fail to become ambulant should be allowed to retain the ability to move from place to place with the aid of a wheelchair. Wards should be generously equipped with them and nurses trained in their use.

Independent ambulation is the main objective of the treatment of immobility. Some patients can achieve this with the help of surgery (e.g. for osteo-arthritis of the hip), while in some drug therapy (e.g. for Parkinsonism) makes a major contribution. But all immobile patients need skilled, thoughtful and prolonged professional rehabilitation. The resource for providing this i.e. the trained physiotherapist, is not and will not be available in anything remotely approaching the required numbers. The few we have must alter their role from being teachers of patients to being teachers of teachers of patients; i.e. they must transmit many of their skills to the relatives, nurses and aides who will be with them.

The attack on the Giant Immobility requires little new scientific knowledge but a major review of resources and their use.

INSTABILITY

Many old people fall when no-one is there to see them. Many lie on the floor for hours unable to rise or to attract attention. They are brought to hospital by the police and they cannot give a coherent history to the doctor. If they have broken no bones, if their body temperature is normal, if they have no obvious signs of disease, it is difficult to know where to begin examining them. Most information comes from the history, and there is quite an art in extracting this from the frightened and bewildered patient, but this can lead directly to the diagnosis.

A fall can be identified as belonging to one of the following groups:— Slip; trip; twist; flop; pitch; and the "rising fall".

"Slip" and "trip" falls are the consequences of an adventurous patient's encounter with an environmental hazard. These occur on the whole in younger and more active patients than do the other types of fall (Brocklehurst, 1975), but they indicate defective attention and tardiness of response. Trips and slips are less common causes of falls in the very old. However, when they are asked to describe their fall, they may use the expression "I must have tripped". I interpret this as indicating their perplexity in falling and their failure to identify any alternative explanation; but in fact the use of this expression often indicates a "flop" fall.

The "twist" fall follows a sudden unplanned rotation of the head, as when, for example, an old lady standing at her cooker turns rapidly to lift something from the table. The possible mechanism is over-stimulation of the semi-circular canals with delayed implementation of the righting reflex. A similar mechanism may be involved in those falls which follow rapid extension of the head and neck, as occurs when curtains are being lifted down or light bulbs are being changed—hazardous tasks in which old people should be helped.

"Flop" falls, also known as "drop attacks", are among the commonest and most intriguing types of fall in old age. Typically the patient says that she (for women are affected much more often than men) was walking in her house when suddenly she "just fell". Pressed for further explanations she will say "My legs gave way and down I went". Sheldon (1960), who described these falls, believed that many victims were unable to rise afterwards because of a temporary paralysis of their legs, and observed that this was sometimes overcome by the patient pressing the soles of the feet against a wall. I have rarely been able to confirm this observation, since most of my patients have lain on the floor helplessly, without attempting this manoeuvre; although some, after a period of about half an hour on the floor, seem to have been able to crawl and to pull themselves up on to a chair or into bed. Many explanations have been proposed for these "flop" falls, but there are few hard facts because of the improbability of being able to measure and record what is happening when it happens. We can at present say little more than that there is some temporary disturbance of the highly intricate mechanism of balance whose integrity we normally take for granted. Basic research is needed here, but the urgent problem is the identification of high-risk patients and the introduction of effective warning schemes to avoid our 20th century tragedy of old people lying on cold floors all night long unknown to their neighbours. (Isaacs, Livingstone and Neville 1973). Regrettably, experience with these systems is not encouraging and the growing isolation of the very old is a grave warning of the need for more effective social planning.

The "pitch" fall, in which the patient is thrown forward in a flexed position, is sometimes an early manifestation of Parkinson's disease. The "rising" fall is easiest to identify and to reproduce. The patient complains of dizziness or lightheadedness on rising from bed, chair or toilet and falls. Some of these patients have postural hypotension, either spontaneous or induced by the prescription of anti-hypertensive drugs. Postural hypotension should always be tested for systematically in those who fall. Other patients seem to have instability in their postural mechanism, possibly due to inefficiency of the otilith system. In others the central nervous efficiency has been diminished by the use of hypnotic, tranquillising or anti-emetic drugs; while others are generally weak because of systemic illness such as cancer, malnutrition or heart disease. In some cases falls are attributed to syncope, as after coughing, micturition or defaecation; while occasionally intermittent cardiac dysrhythmia is the cause; associated either with classical Stokes-Adams attacks or with less obvious rhythm disturbances (Livesley and Atkinson, 1974).

Whatever the cause falls lead to fear. This in turn may manifest itself in two syndromes—one in the patient and one in the caring relative. The former I call the "Three-G" syndrome i.e. the Grabbing Great Grandmother: indicating that the patient is usually a very elderly lady, and the insecurity and instability which she experiences after her falls leads her to place trust in her arms rather than in her legs for balance and support. This subterfuge impedes the reacquisition of leg balance and must be resisted, if necessary, by the provision of a walking frame which distributes the body weight over six legs instead of two. The second consequence of a fall in an old person is the "Three-F" syndrome, or Fear of Further Falls, which afflicts the caring relative. Extreme anxiety is set up and the relative is terrified of leaving the house for even a few minutes in case she should return and find that the patient has again fallen. The geriatric task requires implanting a justifiable sense of confidence in both patient and relative. To achieve this necessitates an investment of medical effort and rehabilitation resources on a scale far beyond that available to even the best of our geriatric departments.

INCONTINENCE

Incontinence is the consequence of organic disease in the organs of micturition and defaecation and their nervous control. It is not a symptom of mental illness as the Department of Health might have us believe (see Circular HM.(72) 71) nor is it a "social problem" (although like the other "Giants" it can create social problems). It is a medical problem and a fascinating one too, which the medical profession has been slow to respond to, because doctors are not immune to the negativity which this most humiliating of symptoms induces. Yet incontinence can be investigated and can be treated with as much success, no less, no more than many other more attractive diseases. Brocklehurst's book on "Incontinence in the Elderly" (1951) based on work done within two years of his qualification, remained the sole major publication on the subject until 1975. Today there are only a tiny handful of hospitals in the country where an incontinent old person can hope to undergo adequate investigation or to receive specific therapy, although at any one time more than 100,000 old people suffer from this symptom, and one person in four will have to endure it for at least a period before his death. (Isaacs, 1972).

As with falls, the doctor faced with an incontinent patient, has some difficulty in knowing what information to collect and how to classify it. Table VI, which has been modified from the classifications of Agerholm (1975) and of Hald (1975) is an attempt to provide a simple bedside scheme of management of incontinence of urine. Most cases of vesico-urethral incontinence need investigation and treatment by urologists, gynaecologists and physiotherapists. Most cases of cerebral and extrinsic incontinence require training and management. In between come an as yet ill-defined group, some of whom respond to newer surgical measures and procedures. Sadly incontinence is a labour-intensive disease. It would be naive to pretend that all cases are curable; but to presume that none are displays an attitude of negativism and despair ill fitting a profession renowned for its drive and resourcefulness. It is the daily experience in well organised geriatric services, with good environment and motivation and encouraging attitudes towards patients, that early cases of incontinence can very often be reversed. Unhappily the majority of incontinent old people are at home, remote from the intensive medical and nursing care to which they might respond; or worse still, they are nursed in large under-staffed and poorly provided wards in geriatric units and mental hospitals with no chance of receiving the human resources that are necessary for their adequate control. It is small wonder that most people think of incontinence in terms of pads and catheters and not in terms of educational psychology and neurophysiology. We are yet a long way from the day when the early signs of incontinence in an old person will be looked upon as a medical emergency justifying immediate admission to a highly staffed investigation and re-training unit. Yet when the organisers of medical care look for a major area of human suffering in need of relief, they need search no further than the Giant Incontinence.

INTELLECTUAL IMPAIRMENT

Widespread belief in the inevitability of intellectual decline in old age, implicit in the use of the word "senility", as a synonym for mental abnormality in later life, is daily contradicted by the outstanding achievement of many gifted old persons (de Beauvoir, 1972) and by the spirited vitality of less renowned nonagenarians. Much of the apparent decline can be laid at the door of the restricted opportunities which our society presents to the elderly to utilise their remaining brain power (Meacher, 1973). This is not to deny that many old brains are badly bitten by disease, but to insist that the consequences will be less disastrous when we provide for all old people a social framework within which their brains can operate.

Failure of the brain in old age should be called "brain failure", and words like "dementia" and "senility", with their overtones of hopelessness, should be permanently discarded. In brain failure a similar clinical picture may be produced by many different diseases, some of which can be very effectively treated. The classification in Table VII directs attention towards those conditions, treatment of which will help to preserve Homo Sapiens into late life (Isaacs, 1973). Every geriatric physician can recount tales of abandoned cases of apparently irreversible brain failure which were dramatically reversed following the identification and treatment of a specific causal disease; and no one knows how many treatable patients languish for months or years under the burden and shame of brain failure.

Those residual patients whose brain failure cannot be corrected offend and frighten us by their departure from socially acceptable behaviour. The hazards of wandering in traffic at night, and of tampering with fire and electricity frighten relatives and neighbours. Inappropriate dressing, undressing and excretion shock them; and increasing irritability and aggression strain the stoutest of nerves and cool the warmest of hearts. Tolerance finally snaps, often after years of devoted care; and the "Battered Granny" (Lusk, 1975; Burston, 1975) now sadly takes her place alongside the battered child and the battered wife as a symbol of unbearable strain. Hospitalisation becomes essential, but some geriatric and psychiatric departments still look to one another to shoulder the burden. Joint assessment and treatment units are providing an answer to this difficulty in some areas but they tend to be alerted mainly to deal with the crisis. Brain failure, like heart failure, should come under medical supervision at its first and not at its last stage. The primary health care team should be alerted to its initial manifestations, and geriatric physicians should be given the opportunity to investigate, to treat and to manage this long disease throughout its course, calling for psychiatric help and guidance as required. In this way, the mechanisms of the failing brain can be observed, understood and explained, the relatives encouraged and the range of resources available for treatment and support can be most effectively deployed.

THE PROTECTED, THE DEFENDED AND THE DEFEATED

In the Scottish study, already referred to, my colleagues and I divided the dependent elderly into three groups. First were those cared for in hospitals or residential homes whom we called "the protected". Next came those adequately looked after at home, who were described as "the defended". The third group comprised dependent old people who failed to receive basic care at home, or whose relatives were subjected to intolerable strain in providing care. These were termed "the defeated". The three groups were of equal size. The "equation of dependence" states:—

the dependent = the protected plus the defended plus the defeated.

In the next 20 years the number of the dependent is likely to grow by one-third, in line with the increase in the number in the population aged 75 and over. That is, the left side of the equation will increase by one-third, and so therefore must the right side of the equation. Thus, even if there is a one-third increase in the "protected" and a one-third increase in the "defended" there will still be a one-third increase in the "defeated". But the "protected" cannot be increased since the necessary resources are unlikely to be available. And the "defended" cannot be increased because the people are not there. We therefore must expect at least a doubling of the "defeated", and thus a great increase in the burden of misery to be shared by dependent old people and their supporters; unless we do something about it.

CONCLUSION

The Giants of Geriatrics are upon us, harrassing growing numbers of helpless people, while a small army of doctors, nurses and other health professionals seek to defend them, with inadequate and often antiquated weapons. The concern of geriatric medicine is by no means solely with the four symptoms which I have selected for discussion. But the specialty must justify itself by its ability to control the great epidemic of dependency in advanced life. To do so it has to work out and to teach its own methods. These will build on the traditions of medicine, nursing and rehabilitation that have served well in the past; but in directing himself into less well mapped areas of endeavour, the specialist in geriatric medicine has opportunities for inventing and employing new techniques of diagnosis and management. I see a major task of this new Department as being to define the strategy and tactics, and to attempt to secure the resources, that will be necessary to defeat the Giants of Geriatrics; and to disseminate these new ideas to the health care professions and to the lay public who share our responsibility for the elderly in our midst.

REFERENCES

ADAMS, G. F. (1974)
 Cerebrovascular disability and the ageing brain
  Churchill Livingstone, Edinburgh

AGERHOLM, M. (1975)
 Classification of incontinence
  Urol. Internat. *30* 3–8

BAKER, A. A. (1975)
 "Granny Battering"
  Modern Geriatrics *5* 20–24

BROCKLEHURST, J. C. (1951)
 Incontinence in the elderly
  Livingstone, Edinburgh

BROCKLEHURST, J. C. (1975)
 Falls in the elderly: relevant clinical factors
  Papers read to the British Geriatrics Society

DE BEAUVOIR, S. (1972)
 Old Age
  Andre Deutsch and Wiedenfeld and Nicholson, London

GRAY, B. (1966)
 Home accidents among older people
  Royal Society for the Prevention of Accidents, London

HALD, T. (1975)
 Problem of Urinary Incontinence
  in Urinary Incontinence, ed. K. P. S. Caldwell, Sector, London

ISAACS, B. (1972)
 Studies of Illness and Death in the Elderly in Glasgow
  Scottish Health Service Studies, No. 17

ISAACS, B., LIVINGSTONE M. and NEVILLE Y. (1972)
 Survival of the Unfittest
  London, Routledge and Kegan Paul

ISAACS, B. (1973)
 The fate of Home Sapiens
  in Symposia on Geriatric Medicine, West Midlands Institute
  of Geriatrics and Gerontology

ISAACS, B. and NEVILLE, Y. (1976)
 The Measurement of Need in Old People
  Scottish Health Service Studies no. 34

LIVESLEY, B. and ATKINSON, I. (1974)
  Repeated falls in the elderly
    Modern Geriatrics, 458–467

MEACHER, M. (1972)
  Taken for a Ride
    Longman, London

TABLE IV

Estimated prevalence of "giants of geriatrics" in elderly population of England and Wales, 2001

SYMPTOM	AGE-GROUP	Estimated prevalence per 1000 of age group 1971	Estimated number with symptom 1971 (thousands)	Estimated number with symptoms, 2001 (thousands)	Percentage change in numbers affected
Immobility	65–74	23	97	93	- 4
	75–84	58	107	145	+36
	85 and Over	166	70	108	+54
	All 65 and Over	42	274	346	+26
Instability	65–74	10	42	40	- 5
	75–84	10	18	25	+39
	85 and Over	29	12	19	+58
	All 65 and Over	11	72	84	+17
Incontinence	65–74	12	50	48	- 4
	75–84	34	63	85	+35
	85 and Over	118	50	77	+54
	All 65 and Over	25	163	210	+29
Intellectual Impairment	65–74	7	30	28	- 6
	75–84	39	72	97	+35
	85 and Over	79	33	52	+58
	All 65 and Over	21	135	177	+31

Data in column 3 from Isaacs & Neville, 1976.

· TABLE V

Index of Geriatric Care: United Kingdom

Year	Numbers aged 45–64 (Millions)	Numbers aged 75 and Over (Millions)	Ratio
1931	9.8	0.8	12:1
1951	12.7	1.8	7:1
1971	13.7	2.6	5:1
1991 (projected)	12.8	3.3	3.5:1